Outsmart Cancer
with
Liquid Biopsy

How to Access this Revolutionary
Blood Test for Early Detection

Dr Hector Daniel Gonzalez

Table of content

Introduction

Early diagnosis of cancer – A failing system

Cancer is a disease that affects millions of people worldwide, with a 1 in 2 lifetime chance of developing some form of cancer. Early cancer detection is crucial for improving treatment outcomes and increasing the chances of survival. The best chance for early diagnosis is through screening in asymptomatic people.

However, in the UK we have routine screening for just three major cancer types: breast, cervical, and colorectal. This leaves many other cancer types without recommended screening options.

Additionally, access to even the screening tests that are clinically recommended can be a challenge for some individuals. Various factors may prevent full and equal participation in available screening initiatives.

Approximately 2/3 of new cancer diagnoses occur for cancer types lacking endorsed screening programs. As a result, a significant portion of cancers are unfortunately detected at late stages when treatment alternatives are more limited.

According to a 2022 Health and Social Care Committee report, only 54% of cancer cases are identified early, which is critical for enhancing survival odds.

By 2028, the NHS Long Term Plan set the national target to diagnose 75% of cases at their early stages. However, no improvement has occurred over the past six years, leaving the UK lagging behind nations like Australia and Canada in cancer survival rates.

Unless future progress closes this gap, the committee estimates that a lack of advancement could result in over 340,000 individuals failing to receive an early cancer diagnosis in the UK.

If you are a man younger than 60, the current system in the UK has no screening for you. Cervical and breast cancer screening do not apply because you are a man. For bowel cancer screening you do not qualify because you are less than 60. However, adults over 50 are 13 times more likely to develop cancer than those under 50.

Additionally, statistics show that 11% of bowel cancer diagnoses in the UK occur in individuals under 50. Furthermore, the incidence of bowel cancer has been rising in recent decades among those aged 20-39 years old.

Let us continue with the example of bowel cancer to see the importance of early detection. Patients diagnosed at stage 1 have a 90% 10-year survival rate, while only 10% of stage 4 patients survive 10 years. Stages 1-2 are considered early, 3-4 late. However, only 45% of bowel cancer cases in the UK are detected early.

To have a proper perspective of the magnitude of this problem, remember that 7 in 10 cancer deaths are missed by traditional cancer screening. On the other hand, if you have an early diagnosis, you can expect 4X higher survival.

Therefore, a critical need remains to explore new screening strategies with broader coverage that may facilitate earlier diagnosis across more cancer types, especially for those currently without standard screening measures. This could optimize outcomes through earlier detection.

Under the present circumstances, why not be proactive and participate in the decision-making about your screening? If you were offered a new technology that can identify early cancer while it is still asymptomatic, wouldn't you use it?

This is where liquid biopsy comes in. Liquid biopsy is a non-invasive diagnostic method that uses a simple blood test to detect the presence of DNA fragments in the bloodstream. It is a revolutionary technique that has the potential to detect cancer earlier, monitor response to treatment, track resistance to therapy, and even predict the likelihood of recurrence.

At present, diagnosing cancer often involves invasive procedures, such as tissue biopsies, which can be painful, risky, and in some cases, may miss the target altogether, leading to false negatives. However, the advent of liquid biopsy promises to change all that, offering a more straightforward, less invasive, and potentially more accurate method for detecting and monitoring cancer.

A liquid biopsy analyses circulating tumour DNA (ctDNA) shed from tumour cells into the bloodstream. This approach can detect mutations present in a tumour less invasively than a tissue biopsy.

While direct to consumer (DTC) liquid biopsies are not broadly accessible currently, some commercial entities do offer something equivalent. For example, GRAIL, the company that manufactures the Galleri test, offers the contact on-line of one of their doctors that will do a prescription for you.

In other words, if you do not convince your GP to prescribe a liquid biopsy for you, it is still easy to obtain the prescription from the same company that will perform the test. In practical terms, it functions as a direct-to-consumer service.

An advantage of liquid biopsies is their ability to capture the heterogeneity of a tumour. Examining ctDNA from multiple tumour sites can reflect the diversity of genetic changes across cancer cell subpopulations. This characteristic makes liquid biopsy the perfect tool to guide precision medicine.

Liquid biopsies also allow non-invasive monitoring of tumour evolution over time in response to treatment or during progression. This makes them a promising tool for serial monitoring of cancer recurrence and therapy response.

This book, "Outsmart Cancer with Liquid Biopsy" is intended to elucidate the immense transformative potential of this technology. We will dive into the science behind liquid biopsies, explore their applications, and look at the research and development being carried out.

The impact of this technology in the UK and worldwide is expected to be profound. Liquid biopsies can bring us closer to the goal of personalised medicine, where treatments are tailored to the individual characteristics of each patient's cancer.

This technology could help us turn the tide against cancer by offering a more proactive approach to diagnosis and treatment, potentially saving countless lives, and improving the quality of life for many more.

However, as with all breakthroughs, some challenges and obstacles must be negotiated. These include accuracy, regulation, and implementation issues within the healthcare system. It is important to remember that while the potential of liquid biopsies is enormous, they are not intended to replace traditional methods but rather to complement them, providing another tool in the oncologist's toolbox.

In the following pages, I will unpack all these aspects, providing a comprehensive overview for lay readers and healthcare professionals eager to understand this game-changing technology. My aim is to provide a clear and balanced perspective, highlighting the promise of liquid biopsies while not shying away from the complexities and challenges that lie ahead.

Welcome to "Outsmart Cancer with Liquid Biopsy" a journey into the future of cancer diagnostics and treatment. As we navigate this path together, we hope to enlighten, empower, and inspire you with the potential of this groundbreaking technology to change lives for the better. Let us step into this new era of Medicine.

Chapter 1

What is a Liquid Biopsy?

Liquid biopsy is a rapidly advancing technology that enables the molecular interrogation of liquid samples, usually blood, to obtain tumour-derived information. This technology has revolutionized the field of precision oncology, providing a minimally invasive methodology for obtaining critical molecular information in real time.

A liquid biopsy involves the isolation and analysis of circulating biomarkers such as cell-free DNA (cfDNA), circulating tumour DNA (ctDNA), and circulating tumour cells (CTCs), from the blood.

Cell-free DNA (cfDNA): Refers to any DNA fragments circulating freely in the blood plasma or serum. cfDNA comes from normal and cancer cells.

Circulating tumour DNA (ctDNA): This subset of cfDNA originates specifically from cancer cells. ctDNA enters the bloodstream as cancer cells undergo cell death and rupture. It contains genetic and epigenetic alterations like mutations specific to the tumour.

These biomarkers can provide valuable information about the genetic makeup of a tumour, including mutations, copy number alterations, and epigenetic changes.

The analysis of these biomarkers can help in early diagnosis, monitoring of disease progression, and predicting response and resistance to targeted therapy and chemotherapy.

These techniques have enabled the detection of low-frequency mutations and copy number alterations, making liquid biopsy a powerful tool for precision oncology. Liquid biopsy has several advantages over traditional tissue biopsy, including its minimally invasive nature, ability to provide real-time information, and the potential for serial collection.

Liquid biopsy can also provide a more comprehensive view of tumour heterogeneity, as it can detect mutations and copy number alterations from multiple tumour sites. Liquid biopsy has several clinical applications, including early diagnosis, monitoring of disease progression, and predicting response and resistance to therapy.

Liquid biopsy can also identify actionable mutations, which can guide treatment decisions. For example, liquid biopsy can be used to detect mutations in the EGFR gene, which can predict response to EGFR inhibitors in non-small cell lung cancer patients. This is referred as companion diagnostic.

Companion diagnostic is a test used to help predict whether a patient's tumour has characteristics likely to respond to a specific targeted therapy.

Despite the many advantages of liquid biopsy, there are also some limitations. For example, the sensitivity and specificity of liquid biopsy can be affected by factors such as tumour heterogeneity, sample collection and processing, and the presence of non-tumour DNA. Additionally, a liquid biopsy may not be suitable for all cancer types, as some tumours may not shed enough ctDNA or CTCs into the bloodstream.

Conclusion

Liquid biopsy is a rapidly advancing technology that has the potential to revolutionise the field of precision oncology. The ability to obtain real-time molecular information from liquid samples has many clinical applications, including early diagnosis, monitoring of disease progression, and predicting response and resistance to therapy.

Chapter 2

The Lifetime Risk of Cancer in the UK

Cancer is a significant public health concern worldwide, with new cases and cancer deaths rising yearly. Statistics show that throughout our lifetimes, nearly all of us will either develop cancer ourselves or know someone close impacted by the disease. Understanding the lifetime risk of cancer can help motivate preventative actions to lower the threat.

More than 165,000 people die from cancer in the UK annually, accounting for nearly 30% of all deaths. Cancer is the second leading cause of death after cardiovascular disease. Every year in the UK, around 375,000 people are diagnosed with cancer – over 1,000 new cases daily. The number of new diagnoses is rising year on year.

In the United States, adjusted by population, the situation is similar. Over 1.9 million new cancer cases are expected to occur in 2023. Over 600,000 cancer-related deaths anticipated annually.

Cancer Research UK estimates that by age 85, the overall lifetime risk of developing cancer in the UK is 40% for men and 38% for women. This means 4 in 10 people will receive a cancer diagnosis at some point. However, not all cancers carry the same risk.

Certain cancers have much higher lifetime probabilities due to their prevalence and the risk factors involved. Prostate cancer carries roughly a 16% lifetime risk among men, followed by lung cancer at 15%. Breast cancer tops the list at a 13% lifetime risk for women, while lung and colorectal cancer have almost equal chances, around 5 to 6%. Other common cancers like melanoma, kidney, and leukaemia each have lower but still significant lifetime probabilities.

The statistics clearly show that cancer poses a considerable lifetime threat for people living in the UK. Understanding these risks and taking proactive steps to minimize modifiable risk factors offer the best strategies for lowering one's chances of a cancer diagnosis over a lifespan. However, continued research and medical breakthroughs also remain vital for further progress in the fight against cancer.

The Inequality of Cancer Survival Rates

Cancer survival rates vary significantly based on the type of cancer diagnosed. Some forms of cancer have seen significant improvements in survival over recent decades due to medical advances, while other less common cancers still have poor prognoses. This disparity highlights gaps in cancer research and inequalities in treatment options and outcomes.

Bowel cancer is the fourth most diagnosed malignancy in the UK, following breast, prostate, and lung cancers. Public Health England reports approximately 43,000 new cases annually. The highest-risk age group is 60-74 years old. However, 11% of UK bowel cancer diagnoses occur in individuals under 50. Furthermore, the incidence has been rising in those aged 20-39.

Evidence indicates that early detection through screening significantly improves prognosis and reduces mortality. Patients diagnosed at stage 1 have a 90% 10-year survival rate, while only 10% of stage 4 patients survive 10 years. Stages 1-2 are considered early, 3-4 late.

Despite this, only 45% of bowel cancer cases in the UK are detected early at stages 1-2. Outcomes are notably better for early-stage diagnoses. Screening allows the downstaging of tumours, leading to higher survival.

With more than half of bowel cancer patients still presenting with late-stage disease, there remains an urgent need to improve early detection rates in the UK population. This highlights the potential value of new screening strategies like liquid biopsy.

Breast cancer has one of the highest survival rates of all cancers. The 5-year survival rate is now over 90% – meaning over 90% of women diagnosed with breast cancer survive at least five years after diagnosis. This represents a significant increase from the 75% survival rate in the 1970s. Early detection through screening mammograms and improved treatments contribute to the high survival rate for breast cancer.

Prostate cancer survival has also increased sharply due to earlier diagnosis through PSA testing and advances in hormone therapy and radiation treatment. The 5-year survival rate now stands at over 98%, though survival drops for those diagnosed with advanced or metastatic disease.

In contrast, lung cancer has a much lower 5-year survival rate of 18%, with only 16% of lung cancer patients surviving one year after diagnosis. The poor survival for lung cancer arises from factors including late-stage diagnoses, lack of early detection screening and limited treatment options.

Pancreatic cancer also has an extremely low 5-year survival rate of just 9%. Most pancreatic cancers are detected at an advanced stage and have spread beyond the pancreas. Effective treatments for pancreatic cancer are also severely lacking.

Survival rates differ even within the same cancer types based on age, gender, race, and access to quality medical care. Improvements in survival have been slower for cancers that primarily affect older adults and certain minority groups.

Overall, survival rate disparities highlight the need for increased research funding for less survivable cancers. Expanding prevention efforts and early detection screening for all populations can also help improve survival by diagnosing cancer at earlier, more treatable stages. With continued progress, all cancers may achieve high survival rates and better outcomes for all.

Chapter 3

Current Cancer Screening in the UK

Screening for cancer aims to detect cancers at an early, often curable stage by identifying seemingly healthy people who may be at higher risk. Early detection through screening can significantly improve survival rates and quality of life for various types of cancer.

The UK currently implements organised screening programs for three significant cancers: breast, bowel, and cervical.

Breast cancer screening:

The NHS Breast Screening Programme invites all women aged 50 to 70 for mammograms every three years. Women aged 71 and over can self-refer for screening. The program aims to detect breast cancers at an early stage when treatment is more effective. Despite controversies, screening mammograms are credited with reducing breast cancer mortality by around 20% in the UK.

Bowel cancer screening:

By existing policies in the UK, screening for cancer is offered to individuals without symptoms who are between the ages of 60 and 74, with a frequency of once every two years. Those who meet the criteria will receive an invitation letter to participate in the screening process, which includes detailed information to help them make an informed decision.

If an individual chooses to take part, they will be provided with a Faecal Immunochemical Test (FIT kit) to be conducted in the comfort of their own home. This kit is designed to detect any traces of hidden blood in faecal samples. FIT kit contains clear instructions on how to collect a sample, which is then sent to a laboratory for analysis.

The test results are typically available within two weeks. If the results are positive, indicating the presence of blood, further tests will be required. The individual will be scheduled for an appointment to discuss the necessity of a colonoscopy to confirm or rule out the diagnosis of bowel cancer. The screening program is associated with up to 16% lower bowel cancer death rates.

Cervical cancer screening:

The NHS Cervical Screening Programme invites all women aged 25 to 64 for regular smear tests to detect potentially pre-cancerous changes in the cervix. Women are screened every 3 to 5 years, depending on age. When detected early through smear tests, cervical cancer is highly treatable, with a 5-year survival rate of over 80%.

Challenges for cancer screening programs in the UK

Despite the benefits, cancer screening programs in the UK have faced challenges, including varying participation rates, false positive results, overdiagnosis concerns and questions about cost-effectiveness. Calls have also been made to extend organized screening to other common cancers like prostate and lung cancer.

Cancer screening remains a critical public health intervention to catch cancers when the odds of successful treatment are highest. However, increasing public awareness, improving screening tests and balancing potential harms against benefits will be vital to optimizing the impact and effectiveness of cancer screening programs in the UK.

Variable participation rates

Screening uptake varies substantially between regions, socioeconomic groups, and ethnic minorities. This means some at-risk populations need to take advantage of the benefits of early detection. Efforts are being made to improve invitation systems and boost participation.

False positives

Screening tests can produce false positive results, indicating a person may have cancer when further tests show they do not. This can lead to unnecessary worry, invasive follow-up procedures and higher healthcare costs. Screening programs aim to minimize inappropriate referrals.

Overdiagnosis

Some cancers detected through screening would likely never cause symptoms or death if left undetected. However, once diagnosed, these indolent cancers may be treated unnecessarily, exposing patients to side effects without benefits. More research is needed to determine overdiagnosis rates for different screening tests.

Cost-effectiveness

There are debates over whether cancer screening programs provide sufficient health benefits relative to their costs for the UK healthcare system. With limited resources, tough decisions must be made about which screening programs offer the best value for money spent.

Limited screening

Only three major cancers have organised screening programs in the UK. Experts argue that offering screening for highly prevalent cancers like prostate and lung cancer could catch many additional treatable cases and save lives. However, risks and costs must also be weighed.

Logistical issues

Cancer screening programs face logistical challenges like shortages of specialised screening technicians and endoscopists, limited screening facilities and difficulties expanding programs to meet growing demand. Investment is needed to alleviate capacity issues.

In summary, while the benefits of early detection are clear, cancer screening in the UK must continue to improve effectiveness, increase value, and optimise the balance of benefits, harms, and costs to maximise the impact on cancer outcomes at a population level.

Chapter 4

What is Cancer? Insights into its Genetic and Epigenetic Origins

Cancer is a broad term to describe a group of diseases characterized by uncontrolled growth and spread of abnormal cells. It is not a singular disease but encompasses more than 100 distinct diseases that can affect any body part. This heterogeneous group of diseases have several features in common, the hallmarks of cancer.

The Hallmarks of Cancer

- *Sustaining proliferative signalling*
- *Evading growth suppressors*
- *Resisting cell death*
- *Enabling replicative immortality*
- *Inducing angiogenesis*
- *Activated invasion and metastasis.*

Sustaining proliferative signalling. Cancer cells can grow and divide in an uncontrolled manner. This is often caused by mutations in genes that encode growth-promoting proteins or their receptors. For example, mutations in the Ras gene are found in many cancers and lead to constitutive activation of cell proliferation signals.

Evading growth suppressors is another hallmark. Normal cells have brakes on proliferation that are mediated by tumour suppressor proteins such as p53 and retinabolin 1. Cancer cells acquire genetic and epigenetic changes that disable these growth-suppressing pathways. Loss of p53 function, for instance, removes a critical checkpoint for cellular growth control and DNA damage response.

Resisting cell death is a defining property of cancers. Normally, aged, or damaged cells undergo programmed cell death known as apoptosis.

However, cancer evolves mechanisms to bypass apoptosis through altering the balance of pro- and anti-apogenic factors. Mutations in genes like Bcl-2 disrupt this balance to favour cell survival over death.

Enabling replicative immortality allows cancer cells to proliferate indefinitely without entering senescence. This overcomes the normal limitations of cell division that normal cells eventually reach. Telomere maintenance by mechanisms such as overexpression of telomerase contributes to immortalization in many cancers.

Inducing angiogenesis fuels tumour growth by stimulating the formation of new blood vessels, supplying nutrients and oxygen as well as removal of wastes. Cancer cells secrete pro-angiogenic factors like vascular endothelial growth factor (VEGF) to promote blood vessel invasion and expansion within tumours.

Activated invasion and metastasis enable cancer cells to spread from the initial tumour site to distant organs. This involves altered adhesion and motility proteins as well as epithelial-to-mesenchymal transition pathways that promote cancer cell migration and invasion. Metastatic potential is the hallmark most responsible for cancer deaths.

More recently, *deregulating cellular energetics* and *avoiding immune destruction* have emerged as additional cancer hallmarks. Cancer cells undergo metabolic reprogramming to fulfil their energetic and biosynthetic demands for rapid growth and proliferation. Immunosuppressive tactics develop to circumvent immune detection and clearance.

In summary, the hallmarks of cancer encapsulate the essential biological changes that collectively promote cancer's unregulated growth, survival, and spread. Continued study of these hallmarks will facilitate the design of new targeted therapies to overcome cancer's complexity.

Understanding the Genetic Origins of Cancer

Cancer is a genetic disease resulting from gene changes that control how our cells function, particularly how they grow and divide. These changes are often referred to as mutations. These mutations are what liquid biopsy will identify in fragments of DNA shed from the cancer into the bloodstream.

Two primary types of genes that can mutate and contribute to cancer are oncogenes and tumour suppressor genes.

Oncogenes

Oncogenes are genes that help cells grow, divide, and stay alive. When these genes are mutated, they can become overactive and contribute to rapid, uncontrolled cell division – a hallmark of cancer. Some examples of oncogenes include EGFR, KRAS, and MYC.

Tumour Suppressor Genes

Tumour suppressor genes are like the brakes of a car, slowing down cell division and preventing uncontrolled growth. They also repair DNA mistakes. A mutation in a tumour suppressor gene can cease to function properly, allowing cells to grow and divide uncontrollably. TP53, BRCA1, and BRCA2 are examples of tumour suppressor genes.

Genetic Mutations: Inherited vs. Acquired

Genetic mutations that contribute to cancer can be inherited from our parents (germline mutations) or can arise during a person's lifetime due to errors that occur as cells divide or due to DNA damage caused by certain environmental exposures (somatic mutations).

For instance, inherited mutations of the BRCA1 or BRCA2 genes are well-known to increase the risk of breast and ovarian cancer. However, most cancers are due to acquired mutations that happen over time, such as those caused by exposure to tobacco smoke or ultraviolet (UV) radiation.

Epigenetic Origins of Cancer

While the genetic origins of cancer involve changes to the DNA sequence itself, epigenetic changes affect gene expression without altering the underlying DNA sequence. DNA methylation and histone modification are two main types of epigenetic modifications associated with cancer.

DNA Methylation

DNA methylation typically acts to repress gene transcription and thus can lead to reduced expression of tumour suppressor genes. Abnormal DNA methylation patterns, such as hypermethylation (too much methylation) or hypomethylation (too little methylation), are often seen in cancer cells.

Histone Modification

Histone modifications also alter gene expression by changing the structure of the chromatin – the combination of DNA and proteins that make up the chromosome. These modifications can lead to either transcriptional activation or repression depending on the type of modification and its specific location on the histone.

Epigenetic Silencing

Epigenetic silencing, a process where genes are switched off through epigenetic mechanisms, can also play a key role in cancer development. For instance, if a tumour suppressor gene is epigenetically silenced, it can lead to uncontrolled cell growth. Unlike genetic mutations, epigenetic changes are reversible, offering potential targets for cancer treatment.

Cancer Biomarkers

Biomarkers are biological molecules in the blood, other body fluids, or tissues that signal normal or abnormal processes, conditions, or diseases. In the context of cancer, biomarkers can be used for various purposes, such as screening, diagnosis, prognosis, prediction of response to treatment, and monitoring disease progression.

Types of Cancer Biomarkers

Cancer biomarkers can be DNA, mRNA, proteins, metabolites, or processes such as apoptosis and angiogenesis. For instance, elevated prostate-specific antigen (PSA) levels can be a prostate cancer biomarker. Mutations in the BRCA1 or BRCA2 genes can serve as biomarkers of risk for breast and ovarian cancer, and the presence of the BCR-ABL fusion gene is a biomarker for chronic myeloid leukaemia.

The Role of Biomarkers in Personalised Medicine

The discovery and validation of cancer biomarkers have paved the way for personalised medicine – a medical model where healthcare is tailored to the individual patient based on their predicted response or disease risk. For example, the expression of the HER2/neu gene can predict the response to trastuzumab in breast cancer. The presence of EGFR mutations can predict the response to tyrosine kinase inhibitors in non-small cell lung cancer.

Conclusion

Cancer is a complex disease originating at genetic and epigenetic levels. While the genetic origins of cancer involve mutations that cause uncontrolled cell growth, the epigenetic origins involve modifications that alter gene expression without changing the DNA sequence. Biomarkers are crucial in cancer detection, prognosis, and treatment, enabling a personalized approach to patient care.

Chapter 5

Liquid Biopsy: Revolutionising Cancer Screening

Liquid biopsy, which analyses blood samples for telltale DNA fragments or proteins released by tumours, offers a promising non-invasive method for multi-cancer screening.

How liquid biopsy works:

Tumour cells that die naturally release DNA into the bloodstream. This cell-free DNA contains genetic mutations specific to a person's cancer. Liquid biopsy tests can detect these mutations by analysing a simple blood draw. The technique can also identify tumour-derived proteins and lipid biomarkers in blood plasma. By detecting these molecular indicators, a liquid biopsy may identify cancers earlier and monitor disease progression.

Potential benefits for cancer screening

Liquid biopsy provides several advantages as a screening tool. It is non-invasive, simple to administer and can detect multiple cancer types from a single blood draw. Only a tiny blood sample is needed. The liquid biopsy also shows potential as a screening method for hard-to-reach organs and a means to personalise cancer monitoring based on an individual's genetic profile and risks.

Challenges to widespread implementation

While promising, liquid biopsy also faces hurdles before it can be used for population-level cancer screening. Studies still need to validate different liquid biopsy tests' accuracy, reliability, and clinical utility. Costs must also come down to enable routine screening. Further research is ongoing to identify the most informative biomarkers, improve testing methods and validate results in varied populations.

However, liquid biopsy does represent an exciting new frontier in the quest to catch more cancers at their earliest, most treatable stages. Liquid biopsy's non-invasive and multiplex screening abilities position it as a potential game changer for the future of cancer screening. Though challenges remain, as technologies mature and costs decline, liquid biopsy testing may transform how the UK NHS approach early cancer detection.

The Fundamentals of Liquid Biopsy Testing

Liquid biopsy tests analyse blood to detect fragments of DNA, RNA or proteins shed by tumour cells into the bloodstream. This non-invasive method can help detect and monitor cancer progression, replacing or complementing traditional tissue biopsies.

Tumour cells naturally undergo cell death and release cellular material into the bloodstream, including:

- Circulating tumour DNA (ctDNA)
- Circulating tumour RNA (ctRNA)
- Circulating tumour cells (CTCs)
- Exosomes
- Tumour-educated platelets (TEPs)
- Protein biomarkers

Circulating tumour DNA (ctDNA)

Fragments of DNA containing genetic mutations characteristic of the tumour. ctDNA can reveal information about the tumour's genotype and treatment resistance.

Circulating tumour cells (CTCs)

Whole tumour cells that have broken away from the primary tumour and travel through the bloodstream. CTCs help indicate tumour spread and progression.

Exosomes

Tiny vesicles secreted by tumour cells containing DNA, RNA and proteins that reflect the tumour microenvironment. Exosomes can serve as biomarkers for detection and monitoring.

Tumour-educated platelets (TEPs)

Platelets that interact with tumour cells and absorb tumour proteins and nucleic acids. TEPs are a potential source of tumour markers.

Protein biomarkers

Proteins released by dying tumour cells can indicate cancer's presence, location, and aggression.

Liquid biopsy tests analyse blood samples for these various cellular fragments and biomarkers shed by tumours into the bloodstream. Changes over time can act as a "liquid biopsy", reflecting the dynamics of the patient's cancer in a minimally invasive way.

The Top 10 Benefits of Liquid Biopsy

- Early detection – May find cancers at earlier, more treatable stages.
- Multiple cancers – A single blood test may detect various cancer types.
- Non-invasive – Requires only a blood draw, not a tissue biopsy.
- Can be repeated easily – It is just a blood test.
- Allows for precision treatment.
- Ability to capture the heterogeneity of a tumour.
- Low cost – Potentially more affordable than repetitive tissue biopsies.
- Real-time monitoring – Can track cancer progression and response to treatment throughout the disease.
- More straightforward compared to tissue biopsy.
- Less risky than tissue biopsy

Applications of Liquid Biopsy

- Early diagnosis (Screening)
- Monitoring of disease progression
- Guide precision therapy
- Predicting response to therapy
- Predicting resistance to therapy
- Predict the likelihood of recurrence.

Liquid biopsy tests have the potential to revolutionise how we detect, monitor, and manage cancer through a simple blood test. By taking advantage of the molecular signatures that tumours inevitably release into the bloodstream, liquid biopsy offers an increasingly sensitive view into the constantly evolving nature of cancer.

Comparison between liquid biopsy and traditional biopsy

Liquid biopsy tests analyse a patient's blood to detect cancer markers like tumour DNA and proteins. They have several potential advantages over traditional tissue biopsies that remove physical samples directly from tumours.

Traditional biopsies are highly accurate and provide a definitive diagnosis. However, they only capture a snapshot and may miss up to 30% of tumour mutations. They are also invasive, expensive, and often require follow-up procedures. While sensitive to detecting advanced cancers, traditional biopsies are less effective for early detection.

Liquid biopsies are non-invasive, easier to repeat and can detect cancers at earlier stages through screening. They can track changes in tumour biomarkers over time, offering real-time monitoring of a patient's condition. And they may be less expensive since they do not require surgery.

However, liquid biopsy tests are currently used as screening or monitoring tools. They still need to improve their accuracy and specificity to match tissue biopsies. False positive rates can still be higher with liquid biopsies.

Factors that allow liquid biopsy to detect cancer at an early stage.

- Very high sensitivity
- Detection of a diversity of biomarkers
- Serial testing
- Identification of premalignant cells
- Detection of field effects
- Genomic profiling

Very high sensitivity

Liquid biopsy tests employ extremely sensitive techniques to detect small amounts of tumour DNA or protein biomarkers in the blood. This enables them to detect tumours before they reach a clinically detectable size.

Detection of a diversity of biomarkers

Most liquid biopsy tests analyse multiple biomarkers released by tumours, including DNA, RNA, proteins, and exosomes. The more biomarkers that are measured, the higher the probability of detecting early-stage cancers.

Serial testing

By repeating liquid biopsy tests over time, even low levels of biomarker release that may indicate emerging cancer can become evident through subtle increases detected on subsequent tests. Serial testing improves the sensitivity of early detection.

Identification of premalignant cells

Some liquid biopsy tests can detect circulating tumour cells in the blood that represent premalignant lesions or very early tumours. These precursor cells indicate that cancer may develop if not treated.

Detection of field effects

Some biomarkers measured in liquid biopsies reflect "field effects" caused by molecular changes that begin before tumours actually form. These field effects can serve as early warning signs years before tumours become clinically apparent.

Genomic profiling

Liquid biopsies that sequence tumour DNA can detect genetic mutations that often arise in the earliest stages of cancer development. Finding these mutations provides an opportunity for early intervention.

Liquid biopsies employ a combination of enhanced sensitivity, multiple biomarker detection, serial testing capabilities, and profiling of molecular changes indicative of very early tumour development. This confluence of factors positions liquid biopsy tests as promising candidates for detecting cancers at the earliest possible stages, even before standard imaging techniques would detect a tumour.

Availability of Liquid biopsies

Direct-to-consumer liquid biopsy tests are available but still somewhat limited in availability:

- Several companies offer direct-to-consumer liquid biopsy tests for early cancer screening, including Lucence and Grail.
- To take one of these tests, consumers order a kit online, provide a blood sample at home, and mail the sample back to the lab for analysis. Test results are then provided online or via virtual consultation.
- Most direct-to-consumer liquid biopsy tests are available only in the U.S. and Canada. Access in other countries is still limited, though some companies are working to expand internationally.
- Because these direct-access tests are relatively new, not all doctors are familiar with them yet. Some may be reluctant to order them for patients or unsure how to interpret the results.

Patient empowerment by liquid biopsy

Liquid biopsy technology has advanced rapidly and promises to significantly empower patients in their cancer care. As testing becomes more standardized and results reliably interpreted, the liquid biopsy will allow patients unprecedented insight into and control over their disease.

Its non-invasive nature means patients can closely monitor their tumour evolution and treatment response from the comfort of their own homes. No longer dependent on intermittent tissue biopsies, serial ctDNA profiling will give patients, in partnership with their care teams, a dynamic "real-time" view of their cancer.

This newfound access to genomic data from liquid biopsies aligns well with modern trends of greater patient autonomy and participation in medical decision-making. Armed with objective, up-to-date information from liquid biopsy monitoring, patients can better advocate for themselves and have informed discussions with doctors about therapy choices.

As liquid biopsy becomes integrated into standard practice, it will empower patients not just with knowledge but also options. Early detection through screening applications, guidance on optimal treatments, and timely identification of resistance or recurrence will give patients more control over their care journey and outcomes.

Over time, liquid biopsy promises to shift the balance of power dynamics in oncology, placing more tools in the hands of engaged, proactive individuals navigating their own cancer experiences. While challenges remain, the emerging technologies described in this book indicate an exciting future of more empowered, participatory patient-clinician relationships centred around genomic tumour surveillance. Ultimately, liquid biopsy aims to put patients, not just their cancers, in the driver's seat.

Examples of specific liquid biopsy tests currently available:

- Grail Galleri test
- Guardant Health Guardant360
- Natera Signatera Test
- Pathway Genomics – CancerIntercept Detect
- Tempus Lab's tumour profiling tests
- Freenome Test
- LucenceINSIGHT
- Exact Science – CancerSEEK Test

This list is not exhaustive, and a more detailed explanation of these tests can be found in the following chapters.

Grail Galleri test

This blood test screens for 50+ types of early-stage cancer across the body by analysing DNA methylation signatures in cell-free DNA. It aims to detect cancers at a point when surgical intervention may be effective. At present, in the UK, the NHS is conducting the NHS

Galleri trial in 140.000 volunteers. This trial will be discussed in detail in chapter 8.

Guardant Health – Guardant360

This blood test analyses nucleic acids (DNA, RNA) and proteins to detect cancers. It sequences 73 cancer-related genes to identify common and rare mutations that may indicate a tumour's presence.

However, it is important to note that Guardant360 is not for screening. This test is designed for advanced cancer patients to help guide treatment decisions. For early cancer detection (screening) they are developing Guardant Lunar. Guardant Health also offers Guardant OMNI, a broader panel test for clinical trials and research purposes.

Natera Signatera Test

Signatera is a highly sensitive, personalized blood test that detects molecular residual disease (MRD) using circulating tumour DNA (ctDNA). It is optimized for monitoring treatment response, assessing residual cancer after therapy, and facilitating early recurrence detection.

Pathway Genomics – CancerIntercept Detect

CancerIntercept Detect is designed for early cancer screening in high-risk but asymptomatic individuals. Early detection greatly improves treatment success rates. Patients and those at risk can take proactive steps to safeguard their health and fight cancer.

Tempus Lab's tumour profiling tests

These liquid biopsy tests sequence the DNA and RNA of cell-free tumour material in the blood to detect mutations across thousands of genes. The results can help inform treatment options by revealing a tumour's molecular profile.

Freenome Test

This multiomics blood test detects eight common cancer types using genomic, epigenomic and proteomic techniques. It claims high sensitivity in detecting early-stage cancers and metastases.

LucenceINSIGHT

The standard LucenceINSIGHT test can identify ctDNA originating from breast, lung, colorectum, nose, liver, pancreas, prostate, or bile duct cancers. An expanded panel, LucenceINSIGHT PLUS, also detects ctDNA from acute myeloid leukaemia (AML) and chronic lymphocytic leukaemia (CML) for 10 cancer types under surveillance.

These represent just a few examples of commercial liquid biopsy tests currently approved or in late-stage development. As technology advances, an increasing number and variety of blood-based cancer screening and monitoring tests are expected to become available.

Exact Science – CancerSEEK Test

Exact Sciences entered the arena of multi-cancer early detection (MCED) screening through the development of the CancerSEEK technology. It is a healthcare company incorporating earlier cancer detection into routine medical care. Their liquid biopsy test, CancerSEEK, are designed to detect multiple cancer types at early stages. The test combines the analysis of ctDNA protein biomarkers to improve detection accuracy. The test is still under development and clinical validation.

In summary:

While traditional tissue biopsies remain the gold standard for definitively diagnosing cancer due to their high accuracy, liquid biopsy tests show several advantages: their non-invasive nature, the potential for earlier detection, the ability to track changes over time, and comprehensiveness in analysing multiple tumour markers.

However, liquid biopsies still need improvement in specificity to reduce false positives and require further validation studies before they can reliably replace traditional biopsy methods. They currently work best as an adjunct to tissue biopsies – a screening tool to identify possible cancers requiring a definitive diagnosis via traditional methods.

Chapter 6

Frequently asked questions about liquid biopsy

What is a liquid biopsy?

A liquid biopsy is a non-invasive test that detects cancer-related genetic material or cells in body fluids, typically blood. It can provide valuable information about the presence of a cancer in an asymptomatic individual. This capacity to identify early cancer makes liquid biopsy perfect for screening. The genetic changes identified in a tumour without needing a surgical biopsy can guide highly personalised, precision treatments.

How is a liquid biopsy performed?

A liquid biopsy is usually performed by drawing a blood sample from a vein in your arm, like a regular blood test. The sample is then sent to a lab where it is analysed for cancerous cells or fragments of tumour DNA.

The fact that liquid biopsy needs only a blood test makes it possible to repeat as many times as necessary. Additionally, it is easily accepted by the public as a screening tool. People regularly go to their GP to check their cholesterol or glucose level. Most of them will be happy to check also for cancer.

What types of cancer can a liquid biopsy detect?

Liquid biopsies can detect various cancers, including lung, breast, colon, prostate, and many others. However, the effectiveness can vary depending on the type and stage of the cancer. It also depends on the test used. LucenceINSIGHT can identify up to 10 cancers. GRAIL's Galleri Test can identify 50+ cancers.

The multi-cancer detection of some liquid biopsy tests represents an enormous advantage over traditional screening methods that screen for individual cancers.

How accurate is a liquid biopsy?

The accuracy of a liquid biopsy depends on many factors, including the type of cancer, its stage, the specific biomarkers being tested, and the technology used for the test. While it is improving rapidly, there may still be cases where a traditional tissue biopsy is more accurate.

What are the benefits of a liquid biopsy over a traditional biopsy?

The first and most obvious benefit is that liquid biopsy can be used as a screening, something that is not possible with surgical biopsies. Liquid biopsies are less invasive, reducing the risk of complications and discomfort associated with surgical biopsies. They can also be performed more frequently, allowing doctors to monitor the progress of a disease over time and quickly detect any changes.

Can a liquid biopsy replace a surgical biopsy?

The short answer is not yet. Liquid biopsies generally cannot replace surgical biopsies completely because they have different purposes. Liquid biopsies are primarily used to screen asymptomatic individuals trying to identify early cancer when it is more treatable. A surgical biopsy is not appropriate for screening.

Liquid biopsy can be used to identify circulating tumour DNA. Additionally, liquid biopsy can point towards an organ as the origin of the cancer signals. With that information, your doctor can order a confirmatory test, for example, a colonoscopy, in case the liquid biopsy identifies the colon as the origin of the ctDNA. An endoscopic biopsy will be taken during the colonoscopy to confirm the diagnosis.

For your treating doctor will be ideal to have both perspectives, the one from the liquid biopsy and the one from the endoscopic biopsy. This is because liquid biopsy can capture heterogeneity in the tumour, something frequently missed by the endoscopic/surgical biopsy. That heterogeneity in cancer's genetic and epigenetic signature is crucial to guide the precision of oncological treatment.

If the cancer diagnosis is confirmed and treatment is administered, repeated liquid biopsies can monitor disease progression. In this context, liquid biopsy can identify recurrence after surgical treatment or response to chemotherapy or radiotherapy. In summary, liquid biopsies and surgical/endoscopic biopsies serve different purposes and can be used complementarily.

What does it mean if a liquid biopsy detects circulating tumour DNA (ctDNA)?

If a liquid biopsy detects ctDNA, it indicates that cancer cells are somewhere in the body, releasing their DNA into the blood. This can be a sign of an active cancerous process.

Can a liquid biopsy detect cancer at an early stage?

The Galleri liquid biopsy, manufactured by GRAIL, is a multi-cancer early detection (MCED) test. In a study, the Galleri test doubled the number of early-stage cancers detected with screening. CancerIntercept Detect, the product of Pathway Genomics, is designed for early cancer screening in high-risk but asymptomatic individuals. LucenceINSIGHT is also designed for early detection.

What information can a liquid biopsy provide about my cancer?

A liquid biopsy can provide information about your cancer's genetic and molecular characteristics, how it responds to treatment, and whether it is developing resistance to certain drugs.

Can a liquid biopsy tell me which treatments might work best for my cancer?

One of the main advantages of liquid biopsies is their ability to identify specific genetic mutations in cancer cells, which can help doctors tailor treatment to your specific type of cancer.

How quickly can I get results from a liquid biopsy?

The turnaround time for liquid biopsy results can vary, but it is generally faster than for tissue biopsies. Typically, results are available within 1-2 weeks.

What are the limitations of a liquid biopsy?

Limitations include lower sensitivity for some early-stage cancers, the potential for false positives or negatives, and the inability to evaluate tumour characteristics that require direct visualization, such as size and precise location. For example, the liquid biopsy can detect a colonic cancer, but it cannot tell us if it is in the sigmoid, in the transverse, or in the ascendent colon. For that crucial information to plan the surgical treatment, we will need a colonoscopy.

Is a liquid biopsy painful?

As a liquid biopsy typically involves a simple blood draw, it is usually no more painful than a standard blood test.

Can a liquid biopsy be used to monitor cancer progression?

Yes, liquid biopsies can be used to monitor cancer progression. They allow doctors to track changes in the cancer's genetic makeup over time and detect the development of drug resistance.

Does insurance cover a liquid biopsy?

Coverage varies by provider and specific circumstances. As of 2023, insurance coverage for liquid biopsies is not universal and depends on the type of cancer, the purpose of the test, and individual insurance policies.

Can a liquid biopsy detect cancer recurrence?

There is growing evidence that liquid biopsies can be useful in detecting cancer recurrence by identifying residual disease after treatment. At present, oncologists' most common use of liquid biopsy is to monitor the evolution to detect cancer recurrence earlier.

Detection of recurrence is the main purpose of the Signatera test, manufactured by Natera. Signatera is a highly sensitive, personalised blood test that detects molecular residual disease (MRD) using circulating tumour DNA (ctDNA). It is optimised for monitoring treatment response, assessing residual cancer after therapy, and facilitating early recurrence detection.

Why might my doctor recommend a liquid biopsy instead of a traditional biopsy?

If you are asymptomatic, your doctor might recommend a liquid biopsy as a screening. If you are symptomatic and your doctor suspects cancer is the cause of your symptoms, if he thinks a traditional biopsy is risky or difficult to perform or if the tumour location is hard to reach. If you already have a cancer diagnosis, your doctor can opt for a liquid biopsy to monitor disease progression or treatment response over time.

What happens if my liquid biopsy results are negative?

A negative result means the test did not detect any cancer-related genetic mutations. However, it does not completely rule out cancer. The sensitivity of liquid biopsies is not 100%, and a traditional screening method like a mammograph might still be required for a diagnosis.

Can a liquid biopsy identify the origin site of the cancer?

Liquid biopsies can help identify the origin of cancer by the specific genetic mutations detected, which can be associated with certain types of cancer. This is called the Cancer Signal Origin. Based on the cancer signal origin, the Galleri test can identify the organ of origin in 88% of cases.

Who has access to my liquid biopsy results?

Your liquid biopsy results are available to you and your healthcare providers. The laboratory performing the liquid biopsy will not send your results to your insurance company, employer, or any other healthcare provider without your consent.

How often should I get screened with liquid biopsy?

Annual liquid biopsy screening is recommended.

What is the future of liquid biopsy?

The future of liquid biopsy is promising. With technological advancements, they may become more accurate and reliable, potentially leading to earlier and more personalized cancer treatments. They could also be used more extensively for disease monitoring and to track treatment efficacy.

Artificial intelligence has the potential to turbo-charge liquid biopsy through enhanced machine capacity for discovering meaningful biomarkers, detecting them with high sensitivity, correlating them with specific cancer types, monitoring longitudinal changes precisely and reducing false positives through sophisticated algorithms

Chapter 7

The GRAIL's Galleri Test

Located in Menlo Park, California, USA, GRAIL is a healthcare company that aims to detect cancer early when it can be more effectively treated. Their flagship product, Galleri, is a multi-cancer early detection (MCED) test that uses next-generation sequencing (NGS) technology to analyse ctDNA in blood samples.

Galleri is designed to detect over 50 types of cancer, many of which are not commonly screened for today. This multi-cancer screening is one of the key advantages of this liquid biopsy over other screening methods that screen for individual cancers. The Galleri test is offered for $949 for self-pay customers.

How Galleri works

The Galleri test is a blood screening test that can detect early signals of over 50 types of cancers. It works by looking for DNA changes shared by many different cancers.

It analyses DNA fragments in your blood called cell-free DNA (cfDNA). Both normal and cancer cells release cfDNA into your blood. But cfDNA from cancer cells has distinct patterns. Galleri checks over 1 million places in your cfDNA. It looks for unusual patterns that may signal cancer.

Cancer signal

cfDNA from cancer cells has certain DNA methylation patterns that differ from cfDNA from normal cells. These differences create a "cancer signal" in the cfDNA that Galleri can detect. DNA methylation is a process that cells use to regulate genes. Aberrant DNA or methylation patterns that differ from normal can indicate the presence of cancer.

Galleri applies machine learning and pattern recognition algorithms to identify methylation patterns that signify an abnormal "cancer signal." This indicates that cancer may be present in the patient's body. The strength of the cancer signal correlates with tumour size, aggressiveness, and stage. Larger and more advanced tumours generate stronger signals that are easier for Galleri to detect.

Cancer Signal Origin

When a cancer signal is found, Galleri uses DNA patterns to predict the organ where the cancer likely started. This is called the Cancer Signal Origin. Knowing the origin helps doctors choose the right diagnostic tests to confirm cancer. Galleri's ability to predict the Cancer Signal Origin (the organ where the cancer is located) is 88% accurate in cancer patients.

Galleri is a screening, not a diagnostic test.

However, Galleri is not a diagnostic test. Diagnostic testing is needed to confirm cancer. Indicating the origin helps guide doctors to the right diagnostic tests for that area of the body. For example, if the cancer signal origin indicates colonic cancer, with this information your doctor will indicate a colonoscopy.

Galleri is different from genetic testing.

Galleri screens for a signal shared by many cancers, while genetic tests predict future cancer risk. Galleri analyses your blood at a specific time to screen for active cancer. But genetic tests look for DNA mutations that show an increased lifetime risk. Galleri can be done routinely to maximize early detection, while genetic tests are typically done once.

The importance of early detection of cancer

Evidence shows that early cancer detection through screening can significantly improve prognosis and reduce mortality. Patients diagnosed with bowel cancer at stage 1 have a 90% 10-year survival rate. In contrast, only 10% of those diagnosed at stage 4 survive ten years. Stages 1 and 2 are considered early detection, while stages 3 and 4 are late-stage diagnoses.

However, only 45% of bowel cancers are diagnosed at the early stages in the United Kingdom. Most bowel cancers are detected later when treatment is less likely to succeed. This indicates that current screening and early detection methods are missing over half of bowel cancers in their most treatable stages. Improving early diagnosis rates could potentially save many lives by detecting breast cancers earlier when treatment outcomes are far better.

Sensitivity of the Galleri Test

Galleri analyses cfDNA to detect abnormal methylation patterns that signal cancer. Galleri's sensitivity and ability to detect a cancer signal depends on several factors, including the type of cancer, tumour size and location, and the amount of cfDNA shed into the blood from the tumour.

Some less aggressive or hormonally driven cancers tend to release less cfDNA into the blood, making them more difficult for Galleri to detect. More aggressive cancers release more cfDNA, even at early stages.

Galleri has a high sensitivity for deadly cancers, like pancreatic cancer. This helps minimize the overdiagnosis of less harmful cancers. In a study, Galleri doubled the number of early-stage cancers detected with screening. Nearly half were stage I or II. This suggests that Galleri may increase early detection for some cancers that lack screening options.

The false positive rate of Galleri test is low.

False positives occur with any screening test. Galleri has a low false positive rate of 0.5%. This means about 1 in 200 without cancer would get a false positive result. A low false positive rate can reduce anxiety, costs, and risks of unnecessary follow-up procedures.

How you can order your Galleri test

Galleri is only commercially available in the US currently. The test requires a prescription. You have two options:

1) Ask your doctor to order the test for you or
2) Request the test through Grail's telehealth provider on their website. Download Grail's Patient + Provider guide to start the conversation with a doctor provided by the company.

Who can order the Galleri test?

A licensed healthcare provider with prescription authority can order Galleri. This includes doctors, nurse practitioners and physician assistants.

Recommended screening interval for Galleri

Data suggests adding Galleri to annual checkups can improve early detection. But your doctor will determine the correct interval based on your risk factors.

For whom is recommended Galleri test?

Cancer risk increases with age, regardless of family history. Galleri is recommended for adults age 50+ because they are at elevated risk of cancer. Adults over 50 are 13 times more likely to develop cancer than those under 50.

However, 11% of the diagnosis of bowel cancer in the UK happens in people younger than 50. That means that annually there are 4730 new diagnoses of colorectal cancer in people not eligible for screening in the UK. Furthermore, the incidence of bowel cancer is increasing in the population between 20- to 39-year-old.

From this perspective, if you are 21+ and you can afford to pay $949 for a Galleri test, I cannot see any harm in doing it. After all, it is just a blood test.

Galleri is particularly good at detecting certain cancers.

Based on available data, some of the tissue types that Galleri appears to have higher sensitivity for detecting include:

- **Pancreatic cancer**: Galleri has shown sensitivity in the 70-80% range for detecting pancreatic cancers, even at early stages. This may be because pancreatic cancers shed higher levels of circulating tumour DNA (ctDNA).
- **Ovarian cancer**: Galleri has demonstrated a sensitivity of around 70-80% for detecting ovarian cancers, particularly epithelial ones.

As with pancreatic cancer, ovarian cancers may release relatively high levels of ctDNA into the bloodstream.

- **Liver cancers**: Early results indicate that Galleri has a sensitivity of around 60-70% for detecting hepatocellular carcinoma (HCC), the most common type of liver cancer. Many liver cancers have an aggressive course and shed high levels of ctDNA.

- **Lung cancers**: Galleri has shown sensitivity in the 50-70% range for detecting lung cancers, depending on the specific type. Non-small cell lung cancers appear to release more ctDNA and thus have higher detectability.

- **Colorectal cancers**: Galleri has demonstrated a sensitivity of around 60-70% for detecting colorectal cancers, particularly at later stages. Colorectal cancers tend to shed moderate to high levels of ctDNA that Galleri can detect.

Galleri generally appears to have higher sensitivity for tissue types that progress more aggressively and shed relatively high levels of ctDNA, such as pancreatic, ovarian, liver, lung, and colorectal cancers. These cancers generate stronger cancer signals that Galleri can more readily detect.

Cancers that are more difficult for Galleri to detect

Based on available information, some examples of cancers that tend to be more difficult for the Galleri test to detect include:

- **Thyroid cancer**: Thyroid cancers are often slow-growing and less aggressive. They shed less cell-free DNA (cfDNA) into the bloodstream, making them harder for liquid biopsy tests like Galleri to detect.

- **Prostate cancer**: Many prostate cancers, especially early-stage ones, progress slowly. They also tend to release lower levels of cfDNA, particularly in patients with lower prostate-specific antigen (PSA) levels. This limits Galleri's ability to detect these prostate cancers.

- **Low-grade tumours**: Less aggressive and lower-grade tumours generally tend to shed less cfDNA. They generate weaker cancer signals that Galleri may miss, particularly at early stages.

- **Hormonally driven cancers**: Cancers fuelled by hormones, like some breast and endometrial cancers, often have indolent behaviour. They release less cfDNA and generate weaker signals that Galleri has more difficulty detecting.
- **Early-stage cancers**: Galleri appears to have higher sensitivity for more advanced-stage cancers due to stronger cancer signals. It seems to have lower sensitivity for detecting the smallest, earliest-stage cancers that represent the greatest opportunity for cure.
- **Certain tissue types**: Based on Galleri's performance data, it appears to have varying sensitivity across different tissue types. Some tissue-specific cancers may be more challenging for Galleri to detect than others.

However, these are generalizations, and Galleri can detect some thyroid, prostate, and other cancers. The factors above indicate that certain types of cancers are more challenging for Galleri – and liquid biopsy tests in general – due to lower levels of circulating tumour DNA.

How accurate is the Galleri test?

The Galleri blood test from Grail claims to detect over 50 types of cancer with a high level of accuracy, especially in the early stages. However, we need more rigorous and peer-reviewed studies to determine its actual accuracy for detecting various cancers.

Grail cites clinical studies showing the test can detect cancers with a sensitivity (ability to identify positive results correctly) ranging from 76% to 98% and a specificity (ability to correctly identify negative results) of over 99%.

However, larger, prospective studies in asymptomatic individuals are needed to determine the true false positive and false negative rates for each cancer type when the test is used as a screening tool. To answer these questions, the NHS Galleri Trial is ongoing in the UK. The NHS Galleri Trial will be discussed in detail in the next chapter.

Galleri is recommended to be used in addition to established screening tests.

Screening tests like mammograms have proven to lower cancer deaths. Galleri does not detect all cancers. And screening tests like mammograms should be used to maximize early detection. In a study, Galleri doubled the number of screen-detected cancers. This shows it can find more cancers missed by standard screening.

Some notes of caution

- Galleri does not detect all cancers and should be used in addition to – not instead of – other recommended screening tests.
- Results should be interpreted by a doctor based on your history and symptoms.
- A "No Cancer Signal Detected" result does not rule out cancer.
- A "Cancer Signal Detected" result requires confirmatory diagnostic tests to confirm cancer.
- False positive and negative results can occur.
- The Galleri test should not be used if you are: under 21, pregnant, or currently undergoing cancer treatment.
- Galleri is not currently included in screening guidelines.

Confirmatory diagnostic tests required for a "Cancer Signal Detected" result.

- When Galleri detects a cancer signal in a patient's blood, further diagnostic testing is needed to confirm whether cancer is present. A Galleri result alone is not sufficient to diagnose cancer.
- If Galleri predicts a Cancer Signal Origin (likely tissue or organ of origin), that information can help guide which confirmatory tests to perform first. But multiple tests may still be required depending on the clinical scenario.

Common confirmatory tests may include:

- Imaging studies like CT scans, MRI scans, mammograms, and ultrasounds

- Endoscopic procedures like colonoscopies
- Tissue biopsies of suspected tumours or lesions
- The specific tests chosen will depend on Galleri's Cancer Signal Origin prediction(s) and other factors like a patient's symptoms, risk factors and medical history.
- Even if diagnostic tests do not initially find any cancer, it does not rule out the possibility of cancer. Galleri may have detected a very early or small tumour that diagnostic tests could not yet detect.
- Patients with a "Cancer Signal Detected" result should follow up with their healthcare provider to determine the appropriate next steps, including repeat testing or intensified screening.

Conclusion

A wide range of imaging tests, endoscopic procedures, and tissue biopsies may be required to confirm or rule out cancer following a positive Galleri result. Galleri's Cancer Signal Origin information can help prioritize which diagnostic tests to start with but does not replace the need for standard diagnostic workup through established medical procedures.

Chapter 8

The NHS Galleri Test Trial: Liquid Biopsy in the UK Health System

NHS England has developed a novel public-private partnership with GRAIL to test and use their Galleri genomic cancer screening test. The goal is to expediently incorporate the assay into widespread clinical practice pending evidence from ongoing research.

The NHS is currently conducting the Galleri test trial – the UK's largest liquid biopsy study – to evaluate this new blood test that screens for 50 types of cancer. The trial aims to determine whether the Galleri test from Grail can facilitate earlier cancer diagnosis and improve patient outcomes within the NHS.

How the Galleri test works

The Galleri test analyses a blood sample for methylation signatures – changes in DNA that can indicate the presence of cancer. The test screens for abnormal methylation patterns across more than 700 genes to reveal early-stage cancers across multiple organ sites from a single blood draw.

The NHS Trial.

- 140,000 participants: The trial recruited 140,000 participants aged 50-77 with no apparent cancer symptoms.
- 6-month screenings: Participants will have their blood drawn for the Grail test every 6 months for 3 years to detect changes over time that may indicate emerging cancers.
- Randomised design: Participants will be randomly assigned to receive Galleri test results or act as a control group receiving standard NHS care. This will help evaluate if the test improves cancer detection rates.

Potential benefits

- Multi-cancer screening: The test may identify multiple cancer types that are currently difficult to detect early through existing screening programs.
- Earlier detection: Liquid biopsy detection of methylation changes could find cancers at an earlier, more treatable stage than traditional diagnostic methods.
- Reduce NHS costs: Earlier diagnosis could reduce health service costs associated with more advanced cancers by facilitating effective interventions.

Challenges to address

- Test accuracy: The trial aims to determine the actual accuracy of the Galleri test in detecting early cancers while limiting false positive results.
- Unintended harms: The consequences of identifying potentially indolent cancers that would not become life-threatening must be weighed.
- Clinical follow-up: The NHS must be prepared for the clinical follow-up required for participants who receive abnormal test results.

The NHS approach to cancer after the Galleri test

The Galleri test could transform the NHS approach to cancer screening if shown to be effective. However, a large-scale trial is needed to provide robust real-world evidence on test performance, clinical outcomes, resource utilisation and ethical considerations before liquid biopsy enters mainstream medical practice in the UK.

In summary, the NHS Galleri trial represents a significant opportunity to rigorously evaluate a promising new approach to early cancer detection through liquid biopsy. The findings can potentially reshape how the UK health system approaches cancer screening in the future.

How long will it take for the trial to be completed?

The NHS Galleri test trial is expected to take at least five years to be completed, with key milestones as follows:

- Trial launch (2021) – The trial began recruiting participants in June 2021.
- Participant recruitment (2021-2023) – The recruitment of 140,000 participants is completed.
- Initial blood draws and screening (2021-2024) – Participants will have their first blood sample collected and the Galleri test performed after enrolment.
- Monthly screenings (2021-2026) – Participants will continue to receive repeat Galleri tests every six months for 3 to 5 years from their enrolment date.
- Interim analyses (2023-2025) – Interim analyses of preliminary trial data will likely be conducted after 2 to 3 years to evaluate progress and outcomes.
- Final trial data collection (2025-2026) – All participant samples and relevant health outcome data will need to be collected and analysed.
- Data analysis and evaluation (2026-2027) – Thorough analysis of all trial data will require at least one year to determine effectiveness and yield conclusions.
- Trial publication (2027-2028) – Formal publication of the entire trial results, including detailed methodology and outcomes, generally takes 1 to 2 years after data collection.
- The findings will inform the UK National Screening Committee's deliberations regarding future population-level screening programs.

Given the large scale of the study, with 140,000 participants undergoing repeated screening over multiple years, the 5-year timeline for preliminary results from initial participants seems realistic. However, it will likely take closer to 8-10 years for the full NHS Galleri trial to be completed with complete data analysis, follow-up, and formal publication of conclusions.

Extensive biomarker studies typically require considerable time for a thorough evaluation.

Ways to stay updated on the progress of the NHS Galleri test trial:

- NHS Website – The NHS currently has an overview page about the Galleri trial that provides background, details on how to participate, and information about the liquid biopsy test. Over time, the NHS may update the trial's progress and outcomes on this page.
- Trial Registry – Clinical trials are often registered with public databases like clinicaltrials.gov that provide basic information on the study and are updated as the trial proceeds with summary results once completed. The Galleri trial is registered there under the identifier NCT04869269.
- Press Releases – Companies involved in the trial, like Grail which developed the Galleri test, sometimes issue press releases at significant milestones to update trial progress and preliminary findings. These can be found on their websites or in news reports.

Chapter 9

Other companies offering Liquid biopsy.

Traditionally ordered by healthcare providers, some liquid biopsy tests have become available directly to consumers online without a prescription. As DTC genetic testing becomes more commonplace, consumers must understand the landscape. While several companies offer liquid biopsy tests, FDA approval and test cost are important considerations.

Remembering that a doctor's input is vital when interpreting these complex results and making treatment decisions is crucial. As this field continues to evolve, we can expect to see more options for patients, improvements in technology, and, hopefully, better outcomes in the fight against cancer.

Direct-to-Consumer Liquid Biopsy Companies

In recent years, the healthcare industry has significantly shifted towards personalized medicine, with liquid biopsies emerging as a groundbreaking technology. These non-invasive tests use a simple blood sample to detect genetic mutations and alterations, offering invaluable insights into the genetic makeup of various cancers. This information can guide treatment decisions and monitor disease progression.

Several companies offer direct-to-consumer (DTC) liquid biopsy tests, but not all have Food and Drug Administration (FDA) approval.

To obtain a liquid biopsy test, the process is usually straightforward. A doctor's order is typically required, after which a sample collection kit is sent to the patient or the medical facility. The patient's blood sample is then sent back to the lab for analysis, and the results are delivered to the physician and the patient within a couple of weeks.

While direct to consumer (DTC) liquid biopsies are not broadly accessible currently, some commercial entities do offer the service. For example,

GRAIL, the company that manufactures the Galleri test, offers the contact on-line of one of their doctors that will do a prescription for you.

In summary, if you do not convince your GP to prescribe a liquid biopsy for you, don't worry, it is still easy to obtain the prescription from the same company that will perform the test. In practical terms, it functions as a direct-to-consumer service. Having said that, the ideal way is to conduct the entire process in partnership with your doctor.

Pathway Genomics

CancerIntercept Tests

Pathway Genomics, a global precision diagnostics company, offers CancerIntercept, their first liquid biopsy test for early cancer detection and monitoring, starting at $299. CancerIntercept detects mutations commonly associated with lung, breast, ovarian, colorectal cancers, and melanoma, as well as less frequent mutations in other cancer types.

CancerIntercept Detect is designed for early cancer screening in high-risk but asymptomatic individuals. Early detection greatly improves treatment success rates. Patients and those at risk can take proactive steps to safeguard their health and fight cancer.

CancerIntercept Monitor monitors patients with active or previously diagnosed cancer. Both tests identify small DNA fragments shed from tumours into blood, analysing 96 frequent mutations across nine cancer genes.

CancerIntercept Monitor supplements more invasive biopsies and scans by serially monitoring cancer response, progression, and recurrence via liquid biopsy. It also offers personalized clinical trial matching for later-stage patients. Rising tumour DNA may indicate progression before imaging evidence. The tests may also detect new resistance mutations over time.

Testing is initiated through patients' physicians or Pathway's referral network. A discounted subscription supports repeat monitoring. Pathway streamlines the process from order to results delivery in 2-3 weeks via physicians, mobile phlebotomists, and oncology support. All positive results are discussed with treating physicians.

Since 2008, Pathway Genomics has delivered innovative healthcare solutions as a leader in commercial precision diagnostics. Their program with IBM Watson is the first to merge AI, genetics, and personalized health information. Pathway's CLIA/CAP laboratory provides actionable precision care information globally across cancer, cardiac, inherited and drug response testing.

Lucence

LucenceINSIGHT

LucenceINSIGHT leverages unique technology to amplify and detect circulating tumour DNA (ctDNA) fragments released from cancer cells into the bloodstream. Proprietary algorithms then analyse the ctDNA signal profile using machine learning techniques. This cross-examination provides insights into the potential origin of the detected ctDNA.

The standard LucenceINSIGHT test can identify ctDNA originating from breast, lung, colorectum, nose, liver, pancreas, prostate, or bile duct cancers. An expanded panel, LucenceINSIGHT PLUS, also detects ctDNA from acute myeloid leukaemia (AML) and chronic lymphocytic leukaemia (CML) for 10 cancer types under surveillance.

By amplification and computational analysis of ctDNA in a blood sample, LucenceINSIGHT identifies actionable signs of cancer without more invasive tissue biopsy. The test aims to indicate the primary tumour site to guide follow-up diagnostic efforts.

LucenceINSIGHT Intended Use and Recommendations

LucenceINSIGHT is designed for screening asymptomatic individuals to detect potential cancer signals through blood-based analysis of circulating tumour DNA (ctDNA).

For patients with a previous cancer history, results from LucenceINSIGHT may be altered. Any past medical history of cancer could influence ctDNA detection and interpretation of potential tumour origin insights.

In such cases of known prior malignancy, Lucence recommends using their other liquid biopsy test, LiquidHALLMARK®, instead of Lucence INSIGHT.

LiquidHALLMARK® is optimized to monitor disease status through sensitive profiling of mutation markers in both ctDNA and ctRNA over time. It provides personalized, longitudinal surveillance and therapy guidance tailored for cancer patients.

Therefore, if you have a history of cancer, LiquidHALLMARK® is the more suitable liquid biopsy option compared to LucenceINSIGHT's screening-focused intended use for asymptomatic individuals.

Lucence LiquidHALLMARK

LiquidHALLMARK from Lucence is a next-generation sequencing assay that sensitively profiles both cell-free DNA and RNA in blood to characterize a patient's unique cancer. With a simple blood draw, LiquidHALLMARK provides valuable information to guide cancer management when tissue biopsy is limited or not possible.

The test analyses 80 genes for ctDNA mutations and 10 for fusions, detecting variants down to 0.1%. Additionally, 36 gene fusions can be assessed through ctRNA analysis (US only; investigational). LiquidHALLMARK targets genes clinically relevant for 15 common cancers like lung, breast, and colon.

Beyond initial therapy selection, LiquidHALLMARK aids physicians in monitoring treatment response over time by detecting emerging mutations that drive resistance. Its high sensitivity identifies more actionable alterations to personalize care decisions across the cancer journey.

Gene fusions guide matched targeted therapies, so LiquidHALLMARK's multi-omics approach increases clinically meaningful findings to optimize care and clinical trial matching.

1) Lucence partners globally with biopharmaceutical companies across the development pipeline from discovery through companion

diagnostics. A companion diagnostic is a test used to help predict whether a patient's tumour has characteristics likely to respond to a specific targeted therapy.

AmpliMark, Lucence's proprietary error-correction technology, improves the detection of mutation types like SNVs, indels, CNVs, fusions and MSI using unique molecular barcodes.

Freenome

Cancer can be solved through early detection, the most treatable stage. Freenome is developing accessible blood tests to help everyone get screened. Their tests detect the body's earliest warning signs using a multi-omics platform analysing tumour and non-tumour signals.

The first blood test developed by Freenome detects colorectal cancer (CRC), the second deadliest cancer in the U.S. Though CRC is one of the most treatable when detected early, more than 1/3 of eligible people do not get screened. The Freenome CRC blood test aims to improve this by making screening easier to access and detect CRC earlier. It is being validated through PREEMPT CRC®, the largest study of its kind.

Though CRC is just one cancer they aim to detect, there are over 100 cancers, each requiring different detection, diagnosis, and treatment. Freenome thus tailors their multi-cancer screening tests to cancer signals, screening goals and patient pathways for optimal outcomes.

The Vallania Study and **The Sanderson Study** are enrolling patients across the U.S. Examining proteins, RNA, DNA, and other biomarkers reveal tumour and non-tumour biological signals that differ by cancer stage and type. This holistic analysis using multiple levels of biology enables the detection of early cancer indications.

PREEMPT CRC was conducted across 200 study sites in urban and rural communities across the U.S. It enrolled 40,000 participants from diverse racial, ethnic, and socioeconomic backgrounds to ensure product effectiveness for all.

The Vallania Study aims to enrol 5,400 individuals aged 30 and older by providing blood samples. The goal is to develop blood tests that accurately detect cancer in its earliest stages in a patient-friendly manner. The study honours a Freenome scientist's mother who battled pancreatic cancer. The Sanderson Study also involves blood sample collection to develop blood tests for accurate, convenient, and patient-friendly cancer screening.

Providing blood samples in clinical studies can help detect cancer early through blood tests—earlier detection results in higher survival rates – up to 8 times higher for some cancers.

PREEMPT CRC Study

Freenome announced the completion of enrolment for PREEMPT CRC, their large study validating a blood test for early detection of colorectal cancer (CRC). PREEMPT CRC builds on data showing the test can detect early-stage CRC with 94% sensitivity and 94% specificity using a standard blood draw. The test combines tumour and non-tumour blood signals with machine learning.

Launched in May 2020, PREEMPT CRC enrolled over 35,000 racially, ethnically, and socioeconomically diverse participants. The study continued enrolment despite the pandemic through a hybrid virtual and traditional recruitment strategy. Participants were enrolled at over 200 study sites, including community hospitals, health systems, clinics, academic centres and through home phlebotomy. Eligible patients could enrol through their providers.

Early data shows the study includes approximately 11.3% Black and 10.3% Hispanic participants. PREEMPT CRC aimed to be representative of the U.S. population, enrolling participants across genders, ethnicities, incomes, and insurance types across all states. With diverse representation, the study will evaluate test performance across populations to support regulatory filings and guideline inclusion to enable accessible CRC screening.

Natera

Signatera Test

Signatera is a highly sensitive, personalized blood test that detects molecular residual disease (MRD) using circulating tumour DNA (ctDNA). It is optimized for monitoring treatment response, assessing residual cancer after therapy, and facilitating early recurrence detection.

Signatera's use of liquid biopsy to detect genomic changes provides an additional monitoring tool that could potentially identify responses or progression earlier than waiting for changes to appear on imaging. However, more data would be needed to quantify its performance advantages.

Medicare covers Signatera for ongoing monitoring in colorectal, muscle-invasive bladder, or stage IIb breast cancer patients. It can also track responses to immunotherapy in patients with any solid tumour type.

What Makes Signatera Unique

Unlike other liquid biopsy tests, Signatera is specifically intended to sensitively identify small amounts of remaining disease rather than as an early screening tool or finding targetable mutations. It is uniquely tailored for each individual using their tumour's distinctive genetic profile to track MRD over time precisely.

How the Test Works

A single analysis of blood and tissue maps a patient's unique tumour mutations. Then dedicated MRD testing tracks those markers serially to pinpoint molecular recurrence risks. Understanding results from this highly tailored approach better inform care.

No two cancers are alike. Signatera is personalized to detect the specific genetic markers of an individual's tumour. Getting earlier insight into ongoing disease can better inform treatment decisions.

Waiting between scans can cause anxiety for some. Signatera provides extra surveillance to help address questions about treatment effectiveness or recurrence risk.

Empowerment Through Information

For one-man, regular Signatera testing allowed him to play a more proactive role in his healthcare. Having insight into molecular changes gives patients strength and control over their situation.

Validated Performance Across Cancer Types

Signatera accurately monitors disease in multiple contexts. Learn how it fits in your care plan based on your diagnosis and treatment course. This unique blood test hinges on analysing an individual's tumour DNA profile. It detects smaller amounts of residual disease sooner than standard methods to guide clinical decision-making.

Signatera is covered by Medicare.

Medicare covers Signatera for monitoring disease progression, recurrence, or relapse in:

- Colorectal cancer (CRC)
- Muscle invasive bladder cancer (MIBC)
- Stage IIb breast cancer
- Response to immune checkpoint inhibitor (ICI) therapy in any solid tumour

Signatera can be used for monitoring other types of cancer.

Signatera could potentially be used to monitor other types of solid tumours beyond colorectal, bladder, and breast cancer.

- Signatera is validated in multiple cancer types, not just the three mentioned.
- It can track responses to immunotherapy in patients with any solid tumour type, not limited to certain cancers.

Signatera tracks responses to immunotherapy in patients with solid tumours

- Medicare covers Signatera for "Monitoring of response to immune-checkpoint inhibitor (ICI) therapy for patients with any solid tumour."

- ICI therapy, or immune-checkpoint inhibitor therapy, refers to immunotherapy medications that help the immune system attack cancer cells more effectively.
- By detecting circulating tumour DNA (ctDNA) in blood samples, Signatera can monitor how effectively the ICI therapy reduces the tumour genetic markers over time.
- Rising or stable ctDNA levels could indicate the tumour is resisting treatment or the immunotherapy is not working as expected. Decreasing ctDNA levels would suggest a positive response.
- This molecular tracking allows clinicians to monitor treatment effectiveness earlier than standard imaging alone. It provides a more sensitive indicator of the tumour's response on a cellular level.
- For patients undergoing ICI therapy, Signatera thus serves as a tool to personalize and optimize immunotherapy based on the molecular changes it detects throughout the treatment course.

In summary, it leverages ctDNA detection to track how well a patient's tumour responds to immunotherapy medications to catch signs of resistance or progression sooner.

How Signatera compares to standard imaging techniques?

- Signatera is described as able to detect cancer recurrence or residual disease earlier than the standard of care tools.
- For patients on immunotherapy, Signatera can help monitor the effectiveness of your treatment.
- This implies it may provide a more sensitive assessment of treatment response than standard techniques alone.
- By detecting circulating tumour DNA, it can track molecular changes in the tumour between imaging scans.
- Standard imaging usually involves techniques like CT, MRI, and PET scans which detect anatomical or morphological changes.

Benefits of using Signatera in the surveillance setting

Based on the information provided, the key benefits of using Signatera in the surveillance setting include:

- It can detect molecular residual disease/relapse with greater sensitivity than current standard-of-care tools. By detecting tiny amounts of ctDNA, it may identify recurrence earlier.
- Using it alongside CEA monitoring can help reduce false positive CEA results, as Signatera provides a more specific confirmation of residual tumour signal.
- Earlier detection of relapse allows potential intervention or changes in treatment plans when the disease burden is lowest/most amenable to additional therapies.
- Patients may experience less anxiety while on surveillance thanks to the additional reassurance of serial negative Signatera tests between standard imaging scans.
- Healthcare providers are empowered with more lead time and actionable molecular data to make confident decisions about the next steps in the patient's care.
- Outcomes may be improved if recurrence is pinpointed at an earlier, more curable stage through the heightened sensitivity of liquid biopsy monitoring with Signatera.

Its high-sensitivity liquid biopsy approach complementing standard surveillance enhances early relapse signalling and decision-making for optimized colorectal cancer patient management and outcomes.

Exact Science

CancerSEEK Test

Exact Sciences entered the arena of multi-cancer early detection (MCED) screening through the development of the CancerSEEK technology. It is a healthcare company incorporating earlier cancer detection into routine medical care. Their liquid biopsy test, CancerSEEK, are designed to detect multiple cancer types at early stages. The test combines the analysis of ctDNA and protein biomarkers to improve detection accuracy. The test is still under development and clinical validation.

The original CancerSEEK assay was studied in **DETECT-A**, the first large prospective interventional trial of an MCED test. Results published in 2020 provided a framework for optimizing a next-generation version designed for minimal blood collection, simplicity, and screening of a broader range of cancer types than before.

The company aims to make early cancer detection accessible through a straightforward blood test, building on foundational research partnerships and the groundbreaking work establishing MCED's clinical validity now transforming patient care.

Designed for routine screening to complement mammograms and colonoscopies, CancerSEEK aims to identify multiple cancer types earlier. CancerSEEK interrogates ctDNA and protein markers to identify abnormalities across cancers, receiving FDA Breakthrough status for pancreatic and ovarian detection. Retrospective studies show high specificity and sensitivity for five cancer types lacking screening.

Cancers that can be detected by CancerSEEK.

A clinical study found that Earlier Detection's CancerSEEK test can detect eight major cancer types responsible for over 60% of cancer mortality in the US, specifically pancreas, liver, oesophagus, stomach, ovary, colorectum, lung and breast.

Additionally, the test was able to identify seven other cancer types that currently have no recommended screening, such as lymphoma, appendix, uterine, thyroid, kidney, ovary, and those originating from an unknown primary site. These results indicate CancerSEEK's potential to detect a wide range of cancer types, both those with established screening and those lacking standard early detection options.

How you can get access to this test

At present, the CancerSEEK test is not accessible to the public, as it remains in the research and development phase under new ownership.

In 2020, Exact Sciences acquired Thrive Earlier Detection Corp to advance the liquid biopsy technology.

CancerSEEK continues to be evaluated in clinical trials enrolling participants at high risk of cancer to validate test performance further. Once clinical trials are completed, regulatory approvals obtained, and real-world clinical utility established, Exact Sciences aims to make CancerSEEK more broadly available as an approved medical test.

Guardant Health

Located in Redwood City, California, USA, Guardant Health is a pioneer in liquid biopsy. Their flagship product, Guardant360, is a comprehensive liquid biopsy test that detects multiple cancer-related genomic alterations in ctDNA. They have 3 products:

- Guardant360
- GuardantOMNI
- Guardant Lunar

Guardant360 is not for screening.

This test is designed for advanced cancer patients to help guide treatment decisions. It is important to note that Guardant360 is not designed specifically for early diagnosis but to decide about the best treatment. For early cancer detection (screening) they are developing Guardant Lunar. Guardant Health also offers Guardant OMNI, a broader panel test for clinical trials and research purposes.

The price of the Guardant360 test is around $3,800, while the price of GuardantOMNI may vary depending on the scope of the study. Pricing for Guardant Lunar is not available yet, as it is still under development.

Guardant360 is FDA approved.

The FDA has approved liquid biopsy Guardant360 CDx which check tumour DNA in blood to guide cancer treatment. Doctors traditionally based decisions on factors like cancer type and spread, but now also use genetic changes found in tumours.

Certain therapies target tumours with specific genetic mutations. The approved test identifies these mutations by detecting DNA shed from tumours into the blood. Doctors can then determine if targeted therapies or immunotherapies may work.

Guardant360 is approved for solid tumours but not for blood cancers. While other approved blood tests check a single gene, this first test for multiple cancer-related changes. Liquid biopsies can sometimes replace traditional biopsies, which are more invasive and slower. The FDA validation means test results can guide targeted therapy selection.

Companion Diagnostics and Tumour Profiling Uses

The FDA approved Guardant360 CDx in August 2022 based on data showing result agreement with proven accurate tests. Guardant360 CDx checks over 60 genes and features predicting immunotherapy response.

Companion diagnostic is a test used to help predict whether a patient's tumour has characteristics likely to respond to a specific targeted therapy.

Tumour profiling – Analysing a tumour's genetic makeup through tests like whole exome sequencing or tumour mutational burden analysis.

Who Should Get Tested?

Profiling is recommended for metastatic patients without standard options or clinical trial access based on cancer type. Liquid biopsies are best if tissue biopsies are complex or invasive. However, tissue is preferred if easily accessible for accurate profiling. Insurance coverage varies, often only if results guide companion-approved therapies.

Chapter 10

Artificial Intelligence and the Future of Liquid Biopsy

Liquid biopsy tests that analyse blood samples for signs of cancer show great potential for noninvasively detecting and monitoring tumours. However, current liquid biopsy tests face sensitivity, specificity, and clinical utility challenges. Artificial intelligence may help address these challenges by enhancing the performance of liquid biopsy in several keyways:

Identifying tumour-specific biomarkers

AI algorithms can scour vast datasets of blood samples to identify biomarkers that best distinguish between cancer patients and healthy individuals. AI can discover complex biomarker patterns and correlations too intricate for human researchers to detect. These AI-discovered biomarkers could significantly improve the sensitivity and specificity of liquid biopsy tests.

Improving the detection of rare tumour biomarkers

Deep learning algorithms can be trained on thousands of labelled data points to accurately detect even minute concentrations of tumour DNA, RNA, or proteins within blood samples. By overcoming the detection limits of current technologies, AI-powered liquid biopsy could identify cancers at earlier stages.

Predicting specific cancer types

Based on analysing large sample cohorts, AI systems may learn to correlate distinct biomarker signatures with specific tumour types. Such predictive models could help liquid biopsy indicate the presence of cancer and the cancer a patient may have. This would enhance the clinical utility of the tests.

Monitoring treatment responses

By establishing personalised baselines and detecting even subtle changes in tumour biomarker levels over time, AI may enable liquid biopsy to track patient responses to therapies and identify emerging resistance more accurately. AI models could also predict treatment outcomes based on blood analysis.

Reducing false positive results

AI algorithms show potential for distinguishing true tumour biomarkers from benign sources of cell-free DNA and proteins that lead to false positive liquid biopsy results. This ability could substantially improve the specificity of cancer screening using blood tests.

Improving low detection sensitivity

One major limitation of liquid biopsy is its relatively low detection sensitivity, especially for early-stage cancers that shed fewer telltale fragments into the blood. ctDNA levels can also vary significantly between patients and over time, complicating result interpretation. AI can help overcome these issues by developing algorithms to analyse complex patterns in enormous volumes of liquid biopsy sequencing data.

By training models on large datasets, AI may recognize subtle DNA signatures that accurately distinguish between cancer signals and normal background noise. This could boost sensitivity and reliability for detecting even premalignant or localized tumours.

Classifying sequencing findings

Classifying sequencing findings is another area ripe for AI contributions. Liquid biopsy often returns numerous genomic alterations of unknown clinical significance. Distinguishing driver mutations that should influence care from inconsequential passengers requires expert knowledge.

AI can learn the functional consequences and outcomes data associated with different mutations to advise clinicians on medical management.

Deep learning may predict a mutation's behaviour, like whether resistance will likely emerge. Such capabilities are crucial as liquid biopsy moves from research into routine decision-making.

Integrating multi-dimensional liquid biopsy results with other patient data

AI's most exciting future application is integrating multi-dimensional liquid biopsy results with other patient data over time. Serial ctDNA analysis coupled with clinical phenotypes has the potential to advance early cancer detection via sophisticated anomaly detection algorithms.

AI trained on longitudinal datasets may identify subtle deviations months or years before malignancy manifests through standard screening tests. Combined with environmental and lifestyle factors, such predictive analytics could empower preventative interventions personalized to individual cancer risk trajectories.

How AI can integrate multi-dimensional liquid biopsy results with other patient data.

- Integrate ctDNA mutation profiles with patient demographic information (age, sex), lifestyle factors (smoking history, diet), occupational exposures, medical history, family history, and environmental/geographical data to develop more individualized cancer risk predictions.
- Combine serial ctDNA, CTC and protein biomarker liquid biopsy data over time with diagnostic imaging scans and reports. AI algorithms could detect subtle changes indicating early cancer development or recurrence before anatomical evidence appears on imaging alone.
- Train models on whole genome and transcriptome liquid biopsy data linked to complete clinical records, including treatments, progression history, and outcomes. AI could discover new biomarker signatures correlating molecular changes with response, resistance, or survival outcomes to guide future therapeutic decisions.

- Link genomic liquid biopsy results to molecular profile databases and clinical trial databases. AI matching algorithms may identify eligible patients for precision trials based on their tumour's mutations, minimizing delays in accessing targeted therapies.
- Integrate concurrent analysis of ctDNA and cfRNA (cell-free RNA) with electronic medical record data. AI could uncover new insight into how genomic alterations and transcriptome reprogramming collaboratively influence disease behaviour and multi-omic signatures of health vs. disease.
- Combine cfDNA methylation profiles from the liquid biopsy with external exposure data sources to better understand the effects of environmental/lifestyle epigenetic modifications on cancer risk and outcomes over the life course of a population level.

Summary

Artificial intelligence has the potential to revolutionise liquid biopsy through enhanced machine capacity for discovering meaningful biomarkers, detecting them with high sensitivity, correlating them with specific cancer types, monitoring longitudinal changes precisely and reducing false positives through sophisticated algorithms. As AI systems are trained on ever larger biological datasets, they may eventually surpass human analysis in maximising the insights gleaned from a simple blood draw to transform how cancer is detected and managed.

Concluding remarks

Liquid biopsy technology has advanced rapidly since its origins and is poised to transform cancer care worldwide. While development continues, the preliminary results of studies using ctDNA analysis are promising indicators of liquid biopsy's future clinical impact. As larger trials are completed, and more doctors gain experience with this tool, its validity and utility will only increase.

Liquid biopsy appears likely to radically change cancer screening, diagnosis, and monitoring method. Its non-invasive nature will make serial tumour profiling safer, easier, and more affordable for patients and healthcare systems. This will enable personalised, up-to-date cancer management tailored to individual tumour evolution.

Challenges around standardization, interpretation of results, regulatory approval pathways, and cost/reimbursement models still exist, but efforts are underway globally to address these issues. With time and refinement, liquid biopsy shows great potential to enhance outcomes for cancer patients everywhere by speeding detection and shortening the feedback loop for treatment guidance.

Overall, we are still in the early days of utilizing ctDNA. But already, the progress made with liquid biopsy technology in just a few short years has been nothing short of remarkable. With continued research support and clinical validation, there is good reason to believe its impact on reducing cancer's devastation could be equally profound. While more work lies ahead, signs indicate an immensely bright future for this groundbreaking approach.

In closing, this book has aimed to provide insight into the science, applications and seminal developments that underscore liquid biopsy's promise as a revolutionary tool against cancer. I hope it has helped illuminate the enormous stakes and transformative possibility that liquid biopsy represents for patients, doctors, and the global health community. The journey toward realizing its full benefits has only just begun.

Glossary

2. Liquid biopsy – A test that analyses circulating cell-free tumour DNA (ctDNA) and other biomarkers in a blood sample to detect and characterize cancer.

3. Cell-free tumour DNA (ctDNA) – DNA from tumour cells released into the bloodstream.

4. Circulating tumour DNA (ctDNA) – See cell-free tumour DNA.

5. Molecular residual disease (MRD) – The leftover mutated DNA from cancer cells that can remain in the blood after primary treatment.

6. Biomarkers – Biological molecules found in blood, other body fluids, or tissues that are indicators of a normal or abnormal process or condition.

7. Tumour profiling – Analysing a tumour's genetic makeup through tests like whole exome sequencing or tumour mutational burden analysis.

8. Whole exome sequencing – Sequencing all the protein-coding genes of an individual's genome.

9. Targeted therapy – Drugs or other treatments customized to the patient's specific tumour profile and genetic changes.

10. Immunotherapy – Therapies like checkpoint inhibitors are designed to stimulate the immune system to attack cancer cells.

11. Checkpoint inhibitors – A type of immunotherapy that blocks proteins made by some immune system cells, called checkpoints, allowing the immune system to kill cancer cells better.

12. Microsatellite instability – A condition where the DNA in specific genes contains an unusual number of repeated segments that can indicate increased susceptibility to immunotherapy.

13. Tissue biopsy – Removing a tumour tissue sample, usually with a needle or during surgery, for analysis.

14. Core biopsy – a tissue biopsy where a hollow needle is used to extract an intact tissue sample for analysis.

15. Companion diagnostic – A test used to help predict whether a patient's tumour has characteristics likely to respond to a specific targeted therapy.

16. Pan-cancer – Related to or affecting many or all types of cancer.

17. Mutation – A gene's DNA sequence change that may alter gene function.

18. Plasma – Yellowish fluid portion of blood that holds blood cells in whole blood in suspension; used to analyse ctDNA in liquid biopsies.

19. Sensitivity – The percentage of true positive results identified by a test.

20. Specificity – The percentage of true negative results identified by a test.

21. False negative – A test result that incorrectly indicates no presence of disease.

22. False positive – A test result that incorrectly indicates the presence of disease.

23. Precision oncology – An approach to cancer treatment that uses an individual patient's molecular profiling to select targeted drugs or immunotherapies.

24. Clinical validity – Whether a test result is proven to accurately reflect the presence or absence of what it is testing for.

25. Clinical utility – Whether a test result meaningfully informs clinical decision-making or patient outcomes.

26. Prospective study – Research that follows subjects over time to find new risk/outcome connections.

27. Retrospective study – A study that looks backwards, analysing records from subjects diagnosed with an outcome of interest.

28. Invasive procedure – A medical examination that entails entering the body, usually requiring surgery or anaesthesia.

29. Non-invasive procedure – A medical examination that does not require entry into the body.

30. Genomic alterations – Changes to an individual's genome like mutations, deletions, and amplifications found in cancer tumour DNA.

31. Tumour mutational burden – The number of mutations within the coding regions of a tumour genome. High TMB predicts response to immunotherapy.

32. Plasma circulating tumour DNA (plasma ctDNA) – DNA shed from tumour cells into the liquid portion of blood known as plasma.

33. Circulating tumour cells (CTCs) – Cancer cells that detach from tumours and circulate through blood vessels are detected in some liquid biopsies.

34. Exosomes – Vesicles released by cells into various body fluids containing DNA, RNA, and protein fragments.

35. Heterogeneity – The diversity of tumour cell subclones within and between primary and metastatic tumours.

36. Clonal heterogeneity – Differences between predominant tumour cell subclones.

37. Subclonal changes – Mutations present in some but not all tumour cells.

38. Temporal heterogeneity – Differences in mutations between biopsies taken at different times.

39. Spatial heterogeneity – Differences between locations within the same tumour or between metastatic sites.

40. Minimal detectable fraction – The smallest percentage of ctDNA in a sample a test can reliably detect.

41. Liquid biopsy panel – A curated selection of genes and mutations analysed in a multi-gene liquid biopsy test.

42. Droplet digital PCR – Highly sensitive method for detecting and quantifying rare mutations in liquid biopsies.

43. Next-generation sequencing – Modern high-throughput DNA sequencing technologies used for liquid biopsies.

44. Ultra-deep sequencing – Highly exhaustive sequencing can detect rare mutations missed by other methods.

45. Concordance – The degree to which liquid biopsy results agree with tumour tissue analyses.

46. Contamination – Presence of nontumor cell DNA in liquid biopsy samples affecting accuracy.

Recommended readings

Nikanjam, M., Kato, S., & Kurzrock, R. (2022). Liquid biopsy: current technology and clinical applications. *Journal of hematology & oncology*, *15*(1), 131. https://doi.org/10.1186/s13045-022-01351-y

Li, W., Liu, J. B., Hou, L. K., Yu, F., Zhang, J., Wu, W., Tang, X. M., Sun, F., Lu, H. M., Deng, J., Bai, J., Li, J., Wu, C. Y., Lin, Q. L., Lv, Z. W., Wang, G. R., Jiang, G. X., Ma, Y. S., & Fu, D. (2022). Liquid biopsy in lung cancer: significance in diagnostics, prediction, and treatment monitoring. *Molecular cancer*, *21*(1), 25. https://doi.org/10.1186/s12943-022-01505-z

Poulet, G., Massias, J., & Taly, V. (2019). Liquid Biopsy: General Concepts. *Acta cytologica*, *63*(6), 449–455. https://doi.org/10.1159/000499337

Yu, D., Li, Y., Wang, M., Gu, J., Xu, W., Cai, H., Fang, X., & Zhang, X. (2022). Exosomes as a new frontier of cancer liquid biopsy. *Molecular cancer*, *21*(1), 56. https://doi.org/10.1186/s12943-022-01509-9

Chen, M., & Zhao, H. (2019). Next-generation sequencing in liquid biopsy: cancer screening and early detection. *Human genomics*, *13*(1), 34. https://doi.org/10.1186/s40246-019-0220-8

Alix-Panabières, C., & Pantel, K. (2021). Liquid Biopsy: From Discovery to Clinical Application. *Cancer discovery*, *11*(4), 858–873. https://doi.org/10.1158/2159-8290.CD-20-1311

Ye, Q., Ling, S., Zheng, S., & Xu, X. (2019). Liquid biopsy in hepatocellular carcinoma: circulating tumor cells and circulating tumor DNA. *Molecular cancer*, *18*(1), 114. https://doi.org/10.1186/s12943-019-1043-x

Zhang, Z., Wu, H., Chong, W., Shang, L., Jing, C., & Li, L. (2022). Liquid biopsy in gastric cancer: predictive and prognostic biomarkers. *Cell death & disease*, *13*(10), 903. https://doi.org/10.1038/s41419-022-05350-2

Raza, A., Khan, A. Q., Inchakalody, V. P., Mestiri, S., Yoosuf, Z. S. K. M., Bedhiafi, T., El-Ella, D. M. A., Taib, N., Hydrose, S., Akbar, S., Fernandes, Q., Al-Zaidan, L., Krishnankutty, R., Merhi, M., Uddin, S., & Dermime, S. (2022). Dynamic liquid biopsy components as predictive and prognostic biomarkers in colorectal cancer. *Journal of experimental & clinical cancer research : CR*, *41*(1), 99. https://doi.org/10.1186/s13046-022-02318-0

Markou, A., Tzanikou, E., & Lianidou, E. (2022). The potential of liquid biopsy in the management of cancer patients. *Seminars in cancer biology*, *84*, 69–79. https://doi.org/10.1016/j.semcancer.2022.03.013

Freitas, A. J. A., Causin, R. L., Varuzza, M. B., Calfa, S., Hidalgo Filho, C. M. T., Komoto, T. T., Souza, C. P., & Marques, M. M. C. (2022). Liquid Biopsy as a Tool for the Diagnosis, Treatment, and Monitoring of Breast Cancer. *International journal of molecular sciences*, *23*(17), 9952. https://doi.org/10.3390/ijms23179952

Lousada-Fernandez, F., Rapado-Gonzalez, O., Lopez-Cedrun, J. L., Lopez-Lopez, R., Muinelo-Romay, L., & Suarez-Cunqueiro, M. M. (2018). Liquid Biopsy in Oral Cancer. *International journal of molecular sciences*, *19*(6), 1704. https://doi.org/10.3390/ijms19061704

Lone, S. N., Nisar, S., Masoodi, T., Singh, M., Rizwan, A., Hashem, S., El-Rifai, W., Bedognetti, D., Batra, S. K., Haris, M., Bhat, A. A., & Macha, M. A. (2022). Liquid biopsy: a step closer to transform diagnosis, prognosis and future of cancer treatments. *Molecular cancer*, *21*(1), 79. https://doi.org/10.1186/s12943-022-01543-7

Cescon, D. W., Bratman, S. V., Chan, S. M., & Siu, L. L. (2020). Circulating tumor DNA and liquid biopsy in oncology. *Nature cancer*, *1*(3), 276–290. https://doi.org/10.1038/s43018-020-0043-5

Malapelle, U., Pisapia, P., Addeo, A., Arrieta, O., Bellosillo, B., Cardona, A. F., Cristofanilli, M., De Miguel-Perez, D., Denninghoff, V., Durán, I., Jantus-Lewintre, E., Nuzzo, P. V., O'Byrne, K., Pauwels, P., Pickering, E. M., Raez, L. E., Russo, A., Serrano, M. J., Gandara, D. R., Troncone, G., … Rolfo, C. (2021). Liquid biopsy from research to clinical practice: focus on non-small cell lung cancer. *Expert review of molecular diagnostics*, *21*(11), 1165–1178. https://doi.org/10.1080/14737159.2021.1985468

Lin, B., Lei, Y., Wang, J., Zhu, L., Wu, Y., Zhang, H., Wu, L., Zhang, P., & Yang, C. (2021). Microfluidic-Based Exosome Analysis for Liquid Biopsy. *Small methods*, *5*(3), e2001131. https://doi.org/10.1002/smtd.202001131

Rolfo, C., Mack, P. C., Scagliotti, G. V., Baas, P., Barlesi, F., Bivona, T. G., Herbst, R. S., Mok, T. S., Peled, N., Pirker, R., Raez, L. E., Reck, M., Riess, J. W., Sequist, L. V., Shepherd, F. A., Sholl, L. M., Tan, D. S. W., Wakelee, H. A., Wistuba, I. I., Wynes, M. W., ... Gandara, D. R. (2018). Liquid Biopsy for Advanced Non-Small Cell Lung Cancer (NSCLC): A Statement Paper from the IASLC. *Journal of thoracic oncology : official publication of the International Association for the Study of Lung Cancer*, *13*(9), 1248–1268. https://doi.org/10.1016/j.jtho.2018.05.030

Barrera-Saldaña, H. A., Fernández-Garza, L. E., & Barrera-Barrera, S. A. (2021). Liquid biopsy in chronic liver disease. *Annals of hepatology*, *20*, 100197. https://doi.org/10.1016/j.aohep.2020.03.008

Ma, S., Zhou, M., Xu, Y., Gu, X., Zou, M., Abudushalamu, G., Yao, Y., Fan, X., & Wu, G. (2023). Clinical application and detection techniques of liquid biopsy in gastric cancer. *Molecular cancer*, *22*(1), 7. https://doi.org/10.1186/s12943-023-01715-z

Chen, D., Xu, T., Wang, S., Chang, H., Yu, T., Zhu, Y., & Chen, J. (2020). Liquid Biopsy Applications in the Clinic. *Molecular diagnosis & therapy*, *24*(2), 125–132. https://doi.org/10.1007/s40291-019-00444-8

Pinzani, P., D'Argenio, V., Del Re, M., Pellegrini, C., Cucchiara, F., Salvianti, F., & Galbiati, S. (2021). Updates on liquid biopsy: current trends and future perspectives for clinical application in solid tumors. *Clinical chemistry and laboratory medicine*, *59*(7), 1181–1200. https://doi.org/10.1515/cclm-2020-1685

Printed in Great Britain
by Amazon